How to Drive Him Wild in Bed

A Comprehensive Guide to Driving Him Crazy in Bed, Mastering the Art of Passionate Pleasure, and Creating Unforgettable Erotic Experiences That Leave Him Begging for More

Cheryl Bach

How to Drive Him Wild in Bed

Publisher: IntimateInk Press

Email: intimateinkpress@gmail.com

This book is a work of nonfiction intended for informational purposes only. The content of this book is based on the author's research, knowledge, and experience, and it is provided with the understanding that the author and publisher are not engaged in rendering legal, medical, or professional advice. The information in this book is not a substitute for professional guidance or assistance. Readers should consult with relevant professionals for advice and assistance regarding their specific situations. The author and publisher disclaim any liability for any loss or risk, personal or otherwise, which is incurred as a consequence, directly or indirectly, of the use and application of any of the contents of this book.

Cover design by IntimateInk Press

Interior layout and design by IntimateInk Press

Printed in USA

Fonts: Google fonts

Image: Freepik.com. This cover has been designed using assets from Freepik.com

For permission to use copyrighted material from this book, please contact the copyright holder listed above.

First Edition: 2024

Distributed by Amazon.com, Inc.

Cheryl Bach

Table of Contents

TABLE OF CONTENTS 3

CHAPTER 1 7

INTRODUCTION TO DRIVING HIM WILD IN BED..............................7

Why a Great Sex Life Is Important in a Relationship 7

Introducing the Concept of Driving Him Wild in Bed 8

Breaking Down Common Myths about Sex 9

CHAPTER 2 13

UNDERSTAND MALE ANATOMY AND SEXUAL PSYCHOLOGY 13

How a Man's Body Works During Sexual Arousal 13

Understanding Male Pleasure Points 15

How to Read Your Partner's Sexual Cues and Signals 16

CHAPTER 3 19

MASTERING THE ART OF FOREPLAY...19

The Importance of Foreplay in Building Sexual Tension 19

Different Types of Foreplay Techniques 20

How to Incorporate a Sensual Massage into Your Foreplay 22

CHAPTER 4 ....**25**

EXPLORING NEW SEXUAL POSITIONS 25

Different Positions, Different Stimulation 26

Discussing Trying New Positions with Your Partner 27

Transitioning Between Different Positions 28

CHAPTER 5 ....**31**

ENHANCING YOUR SEXUAL KNOWLEDGE AND COMMUNICATION ..31

Communicating Openly about Your Desires and Fantasies 32

Encouraging Your Partner to Share Their Desires and Fantasies 33

Learning about New Techniques and Experimenting With Them 34

CHAPTER 6 ....**37**

ADDING SOME KINK AND VARIETY TO YOUR SEX LIFE 37

Introduction to BDSM and Other Kink Practices 38

How to Safely Engage in Kinky BDSM Play with Your Partner 39

How to Keep Sex Life Spicy and Exciting 40

CHAPTER 7 ....**43**

LEARNING THE ART OF ORAL SEX 43

Different Types of Oral Sex..43

Exploring Your and Your Partner's Boundaries.................44

Tips for Mastering Different Techniques............................45

CHAPTER 8 ....**49**

ADVANCED TECHNIQUES FOR DRIVING HIM WILD IN BED 49

Mastering Multiple Orgasms..49

How to Control Timing and Rhythm during Sex 50

The Art of Teasing and Building Anticipation....................50

CHAPTER 9 ....**53**

HOW TO CREATE UNFORGETTABLE EROTIC EXPERIENCES 53

Setting the Mood for a Passionate Night............................53

Creating a Sensual Environment in Your Bedroom 54

Dressing for Success..54

CHAPTER 10 ....**57**

HOW TO KEEP HIM BEGGING FOR MORE 57

Communication is Key...57

Fun and Interesting Sex Life..58

Incorporating New Techniques 58

Don't Be Afraid to Mix It Up 59

CHAPTER 11 ....**61**

ADDRESSING COMMON SEXUAL ISSUES 61

Understanding and Overcoming Common Sexual

Problems 61

Finding Help and Support for More Complex Sexual Issues

....63

CHAPTER 12 ....**67**

CONCLUSION 67

Recap of the Key Points Covered in the Book.........................67

Encouragement to Continue Exploring Sexual Pleasure

with Your Partner..69

Final Thoughts on How to Drive Him Wild in Bed............70

Chapter 1

Introduction to Driving Him Wild in Bed

Why a Great Sex Life Is Important in a Relationship

Sexual intimacy is a critical component of emotional bonding in relationships. A great sex life provides not just physical pleasure, but emotional satisfaction and deeper connection with your partner. It helps to reduce stress levels, build a stronger connection and trust, and maintain the overall health of the relationship.

When you and your partner share a satisfying and fulfilling sex life, it increases your emotional connection, making it easier to interact outside of the bedroom. You will also have a stronger trust in one another which forms the basis of any strong relationship.

In addition, a healthy sex life comes with physical health benefits such as lower blood pressure, better sleep, enhanced immunity and an overall better quality of life. Investing in cultivating an active and satisfying sex life should be a priority in any happy and healthy relationship.

Introducing the Concept of Driving Him Wild in Bed

In order to drive your partner wild in bed, it's important to first understand your own desires and be comfortable with exploring them. This involves having an open communication about your sexual desires with your partner, being confident in your sexuality, and creating a safe space for sexual experimentation.

Cheryl Bach

By providing emotional connection, physical intimacy, and pleasure, you can leave your partner craving more and looking forward to the next time. Your partner will also feel appreciated, valued and loved when they see the effort you put into driving them wild in bed.

Breaking Down Common Myths about Sex

There are countless myths, misconceptions, and taboos surrounding sex that can lead to misconceptions and misunderstandings about sex in relationships. In this section, we will debunk some of the most common myths about sex.

One myth is that sex should always be spontaneous and effortless, but the truth is that a great sexual experience often requires effort, communication, and experimentation. The myth of having to have loud, earth-shattering orgasms can also lead to unrealistic expectations, making it harder to achieve real sexual satisfaction.

Other myths include the idea that women don't enjoy sex as much as men or that certain sexual desires or practices are taboo or shameful. By acknowledging and breaking down these myths, we can approach sex and sexuality with more honesty and openness, leading to a more fulfilling sexual experience for both partners.

Overall, by understanding the importance of a great sex life in a relationship, introducing the concept of driving him wild in bed, and debunking common myths about sex, you will be well on your way to creating a passionate, exciting sexual experience that will strengthen your relationship and leave your partner yearning for more. Remember that the key to driving him wild in bed is to communicate openly with your partner, explore your desires confidently and without judgement, and be willing to experiment and try new things together.

In the following chapters of this book, we will dive deeper into specific techniques and strategies for driving him wild in bed, including tips for improving intimacy and communication, advice on how to master the art of foreplay, guidance on trying out new sexual positions and scenarios, and much more. Stay tuned for everything you need to know to take your sex life to the next level and create unforgettable sexual experiences with the one you love.

How to Drive Him Wild in Bed

Chapter 2

Understand Male Anatomy and Sexual Psychology

In order to become an expert in driving him wild in bed, it's important to have a deep understanding of male anatomy and sexual psychology. The better you understand how a man's body works during sexual arousal, what his pleasure points are, and how to read his sexual cues and signals, the more you can cater to his desires and leave him begging for more.

How a Man's Body Works During Sexual Arousal

Understanding how a man's body works during sexual arousal is crucial to knowing how to turn him on and achieve maximum pleasure during sexual activity. When a man becomes sexually excited, his brain sends signals to his genitals, triggering the release of hormones that cause blood to rush into the penis and the testicles to swell and rise.

This increased blood flow results in an erection, which can vary in strength and duration depending on a variety of factors, including arousal level, physical health, and emotional state. Additionally, during sexual arousal, the body may produce precum, a clear liquid that lubricates the urethra and can help facilitate intercourse.

As arousal continues and reaches its peak, the man will experience an intense release of sexual tension in the form of orgasm. This typically involves rhythmic contractions of the muscles in the penis, pelvic region, and other parts of the body, accompanied by pleasurable sensations.

Cheryl Bach

After orgasm, the man's body often enters a refractory period, during which it becomes less sensitive to sexual stimulation. The length of this period can vary widely depending on age, overall health, and other factors.

Understanding Male Pleasure Points

In order to drive your partner wild in bed, it's important to understand his body and what turns him on. While every man is unique and may have different preferences, there are some common pleasure points that tend to be universally enjoyable.

The most obvious pleasure points are the genitals, including the penis and testicles. Many men enjoy having their penis stroked, licked, or sucked, while others prefer heavier pressure or more gentle touch. The testicles can also be a highly sensitive area, and many men enjoy having them touched, licked, or massaged during sexual activity.

Other potential pleasure points include the nipples, which can also become erect and sensitive during arousal, as well as the perineum, the area between the scrotum and the anus. Some men may also enjoy having their prostate stimulated, either through direct penetration or via external pressure.

How to Read Your Partner's Sexual Cues and Signals

Nonverbal communication plays a crucial role in sexual activity, and being able to read your partner's cues and signals can help you know what he likes and dislikes, what he wants more of, and when he is approaching orgasm.

Different men may have different communication styles during sex, but there are some common signs to look for:

Moans and groans: Many men make noise during sex, and the sounds they make can provide important feedback on what feels good and what doesn't. Listen for changes in tone or intensity to gauge how your partner is feeling.

Body language: Pay attention to your partner's body position, movements, and muscle tension. Is he leaning into your touch, pulling away, or tensing up? These can all be indicators of what he likes and what he doesn't.

Physical responses: In addition to moans and body language, watch for physical responses like changes in breathing, heart rate, and skin temperature. These can all be signs of arousal and can help guide your actions during sexual activity.

Finally, communication is also key when it comes to reading your partner's sexual cues and signals. Don't be afraid to ask your partner how he's feeling or what he wants more of, and be open to feedback and suggestions. By communicating openly and honestly, you can ensure that you are both on the same page and working together to create unforgettable erotic experiences.

In summary, understanding male anatomy and sexual psychology is crucial for driving your partner wild in bed. By knowing how a man's body works during sexual arousal, understanding his pleasure points, and learning to read his sexual cues and signals, you can enhance your sexual experiences and create intimacy and connection that will leave him begging for more.

Chapter 3

Mastering the Art of Foreplay

Foreplay is a crucial aspect of sexual activity that is often overlooked or rushed, but mastering it can be the key to driving him wild in bed and creating unforgettable erotic experiences.

The Importance of Foreplay in Building Sexual Tension

Foreplay is the process of building sexual tension and anticipation before engaging in intercourse. It serves as a way to set the mood, connect emotionally with your partner, and explore each other's bodies in intimate and pleasurable ways. Without adequate foreplay, sexual activity can become routine, unsatisfying, and even uncomfortable for both partners.

The key to successful foreplay is to take your time and explore each other's bodies in a way that feels comfortable and natural. This can involve anything from kissing and caressing to oral sex and more. By taking the time to focus on each other's pleasure, you can create a deeply intimate and passionate experience that heightens arousal and drives both partners wild.

Different Types of Foreplay Techniques

There are many different types of foreplay techniques that you can use to create sexual tension and anticipation before engaging in intercourse.

Some popular techniques include:

Kissing and caressing: Soft, sensual kissing and gentle caresses can be incredibly erotic and a great way to build sexual tension.

Oral sex: Going down on your partner or receiving oral sex can be highly pleasurable and intensify sexual arousal.

Sensual massage: A full-body massage can be a great way to relax both partners while building sexual tension and anticipation through touch.

Dirty talk: Talking dirty to your partner can be a powerful turn-on and create a sense of intimacy and closeness.

Role-play: Engaging in role-play can be a fun way to explore different fantasies and desires, creating an exciting and adventurous sexual experience.

Using sex toys: Incorporating sex toys into foreplay such as vibrators or dildos can add a new level of pleasure and stimulation to your sexual experience.

Bondage: Bondage is the use of restraints, such as ropes, cuffs, or ties, to restrict movement and create a sense of vulnerability and trust. This can heighten eroticism and sexual tension.

Each of these techniques can be used in combination or individually based on you and your partner's interests and preferences. Remember, the key is to communicate openly and honestly with your partner about what you like and what you don't, so that you can create a deeply pleasurable experience together.

How to Incorporate a Sensual Massage into Your Foreplay

A sensual massage can be a fantastic way to incorporate touch into your foreplay and build sexual tension between you and your partner.

Here are some tips for mastering the art of sensual massage:

Set the mood: Before beginning a sensual massage, set the mood by dimming the lights, lighting candles, and playing soft music. This will create a relaxing and sensual atmosphere that will help your partner feel more comfortable and relaxed.

Use oils or lotions: To make the massage more pleasurable, use a high-quality massage oil or lotion to reduce friction and enhance the sensation of touch.

Focus on erogenous zones: Spend extra time on your partner's sensitive areas, such as the back of the neck, ears, nipples, thighs, and genitals. Be sure to ask your partner what feels good and what doesn't, so you can adjust your touch accordingly.

Use your whole body: Don't be afraid to use your whole body during the massage, including your breasts, thighs, and buttocks. This can create a more intimate and sensual experience for both partners.

Explore different techniques: There are many different massage techniques you can use, such as kneading, rubbing, and stroking. Mix things up to keep the massage interesting and pleasurable.

Communicate with your partner: Throughout the massage, be sure to check in with your partner and ask how they are feeling. This will help you adjust your touch to their preferences and ensure that they are enjoying the experience.

A sensual massage can be the perfect way to build sexual tension and intimacy between you and your partner. By slowing down and taking the time to explore each other's bodies in a pleasurable and relaxing way, you can create an unforgettable erotic experience that leaves both partners begging for more.

Chapter 4

Exploring New Sexual Positions

Sexual positions are one of the most exciting, pleasurable, and dynamic aspects of sexual exploration. They can be sensual, adventurous, and downright wild, but they can also be challenging, awkward, or even uncomfortable. However, exploring new sexual positions can provide a wealth of new sensations and experiences that bolster intimacy, trust, and communication between partners.

In this chapter, we'll explore some of the most popular and pleasurable sexual positions for both men and women, as well as discuss how to communicate about trying new positions with your partner, and how to transition between different positions during sex.

Different Positions, Different Stimulation

One of the most significant benefits of exploring new sexual positions is the variety of stimulation they offer. Different positions can target different erogenous zones, such as the G-spot, clitoris, or prostate. For example, missionary is a classic position that allows for deep penetration, while cowgirl/reverse cowgirl can provide direct clitoral stimulation. Doggy style allows for deeper penetration and stimulation of the G-spot, and spooning can provide intimate and sensual contact.

In addition to these classics, there are countless other positions that couples can experiment with, such as the wheelbarrow, the lotus, and the standing 69. The key is to have an open and adventurous mindset and be willing to try new things.

Discussing Trying New Positions with Your Partner

It's essential to have open communication with your partner when it comes to trying new positions. Bringing up the topic may feel uncomfortable or awkward, but it's crucial to express your desires and explore your sexuality openly and honestly.

Start by initiating a conversation about fantasies and interests in the bedroom. Some people prefer a direct approach, while others may feel more comfortable hinting at desires or bringing up the topic in a playful or teasing manner. The goal is to create an open dialogue where both partners feel safe and comfortable expressing their desires and exploring new possibilities.

One practical way of discussing new positions is by sharing images or videos of the position you want to try. This can help break the ice and provide a visual reference to work with. Alternatively, you can suggest trying a new position during foreplay or simply ask your partner if they are open to trying something new.

It's also crucial to respect your partner's boundaries and preferences, and never pressure them to try anything they are not comfortable with. Remember, consent is crucial in any sexual encounter, and it's important to prioritize your partner's safety and comfort.

Transitioning Between Different Positions

Switching between positions during sex is a great way to keep things interesting and build excitement. However, it can be challenging to navigate the logistics of transitioning between different positions smoothly.

Start by communicating with your partner before switching positions. Let them know what you want to try and how you plan to get there. This can be as simple as saying "Let's try going from missionary to cowgirl" or as elaborate as demonstrating the transition step-by-step.

When transitioning, be mindful of your partner's body and comfort. Be careful not to put too much pressure on any one area, especially the lower back or neck, and be sure to provide support where needed. Use lubrication if necessary, and take things slow to prevent discomfort or injury.

Finally, don't be afraid to experiment and try different variations of a position. For example, you can adjust the angle or height of your hips, change the speed or intensity of your movements, or incorporate different types of stimulation such as oral or manual play. Use your partner's feedback to guide you and adjust accordingly.

In conclusion, exploring new sexual positions can be a fun and exciting way to spice up your sex life and build intimacy with your partner. Remember to communicate openly and honestly, respect each other's boundaries, and prioritize safety and comfort at all times. With a little experimentation and an open mind, you and your partner can enjoy a world of sexual pleasure and unforgettable experiences.

Chapter 5

Enhancing Your Sexual Knowledge and Communication

Sexual knowledge and communication are essential components of a fulfilling and satisfying sex life. Sharing your desires, fantasies, and techniques with your partner can create an intimate and exciting experience that leaves both of you feeling satisfied and fulfilled.

In this chapter, we will explore how to communicate about your desires and fantasies, encourage your partner to do the same, and learn about new techniques to experiment with.

Communicating Openly about Your Desires and Fantasies

One of the most significant barriers to sexual fulfillment is the inability to communicate openly and honestly with your partner. However, being able to express and share your desires is crucial when it comes to driving your partner wild in bed.

To communicate openly, start by creating a safe environment free of judgment or criticism. Choose a time and place where both of you feel comfortable and relaxed, and express your desires in a clear and direct manner. Avoid using ambiguous language or expecting your partner to read between the lines. Instead, be specific about what you want and how you want it.

You can also use a more playful approach by incorporating intimate and sexy jokes or teasing into your conversation. This can help create an atmosphere of intimacy and openness that can make your partner feel more comfortable expressing themselves to you.

Encouraging Your Partner to Share Their Desires and Fantasies

Just as it is essential for you to communicate your desires with your partner, it is equally crucial that you encourage your partner to do the same. One way to encourage your partner to open up is to start by giving them positive feedback when they try something new or different in the bedroom.

You can also use a more playful approach by starting a game where both of you take turns sharing your fantasies individually, and then acting them out together.

Additionally, ask your partner about their interests and preferences in the bedroom. Show genuine interest in what they have to say, and avoid being judgmental or dismissive about their desires and fantasies.

Learning about New Techniques and Experimenting With Them

Finally, it's essential to keep learning and experimenting with new techniques to keep things fresh and exciting in the bedroom. This can involve trying out new positions, incorporating new types of stimulation, or exploring different erogenous zones.

Take some time to research and learn about new techniques together as a couple. Watch online tutorials or read books and blogs about different sexual techniques that intrigue you. Then, experiment together and try out these techniques, taking the time to give your partner feedback and adjust accordingly.

Cheryl Bach

In conclusion, communicating openly about your desires and encouraging your partner to do the same can help create an intimate and fulfilling sexual experience that leaves both partners feeling satisfied and desired. In addition, experimenting with new techniques and ideas can help keep things fresh and exciting in the bedroom and improve sexual satisfaction over time.

Remember to approach these conversations with honesty, directness, and empathy. Avoid being overly critical or negative, and encourage your partner to express their desires and fantasies without fear of judgment or rejection.

By enhancing your sexual knowledge and communication, you can build a more intimate and satisfying sex life that is tailor-made for your unique desires and preferences. So don't be afraid to speak up, try new things, and explore the wonderful world of sexual pleasure with your partner.

How to Drive Him Wild in Bed

Chapter 6

Adding Some Kink and Variety to Your Sex Life

Sex can become monotonous and uninspiring without variety. Adding some kink to your sex life can spice things up and intensify the bond between you and your partner, leading to thrilling experiences that leave both of you begging for more.

In this chapter, we'll explore several ways to add some variety by introducing BDSM and other kink practices into your sex life.

Introduction to BDSM and Other Kink Practices

BDSM (bondage, discipline, dominance, and submission) is a form of sexual expression that involves power exchange and can include various activities. It involves consensual acts where one partner is in control and the other is submissive.

Some common BDSM activities include spanking, bondage, sensory deprivation, role-playing, and dominance and submission. However, there is an endless range of options in this practice, and it's important to discuss and explore what works best for you and your partner.

It's also essential to remember that BDSM should be consensual and safe. Any activities involving kink or BDSM require discussion and negotiation before engaging in them. Consent and trust are paramount, and both parties need to feel comfortable and safe.

How to Safely Engage in Kinky BDSM Play with Your Partner

Before engaging in any kink activities, make sure that both you and your partner are on the same page. Discuss and negotiate limits, boundaries, and safe words to ensure that everyone involved is happy and enjoying themselves.

Additionally, it's important to establish a level of trust with your partner. Without trust, it is not possible to engage in BDSM play safely and sensually.

Always remember that BDSM activities carry risks, and proper precautions need to be taken. Make sure to have a suitable environment for these activities and have the necessary equipment. It's recommended to start with "soft" play such as feather tickling or light spanking and work up gradually from there.

Communication is critical throughout the entire process, and checking in with each other regularly is essential. If at any point one partner feels uncomfortable, they should be encouraged to speak up, and play should stop immediately.

Additionally, it's essential to have a plan in case something goes wrong. Ensure that both you and your partner know what to do in the case of an emergency.

How to Keep Sex Life Spicy and Exciting

Adding kink to your sex life is just one way to keep things spicy and exciting. Other ways include exploring new positions, trying new techniques, and incorporating sex toys into your playtime.

It's also important to continue to communicate with your partner about your desires and needs to ensure that both of you are satisfied with your intimate experiences. Don't be afraid to experiment and try new things, as long as you both feel comfortable and safe.

Planning date nights or weekend getaways can also help keep things exciting. Take some time to explore erotic fantasies together, go out and try new things, or engage in sexual activities in new and exciting settings.

Don't forget the importance of physical touch outside of the bedroom as well. Hugging, kissing, holding hands, and cuddling are essential to maintaining intimacy and fostering a deeper emotional connection with your partner.

In conclusion, adding some kink to your sex life can be a thrilling and exciting experience if done safely and consensually. Remember to communicate with your partner, establish trust and consent before engaging in any BDSM or other kink activities, and always prioritize your safety.

In addition to exploring kink, don't forget to mix things up in other ways as well. Keep communication open and honest, try new things, and don't be afraid to experiment with different positions, techniques, and sex toys.

Ultimately, the most important thing is that both you and your partner feel comfortable and satisfied with your sex life. So don't be afraid to explore, take risks, and have fun in the bedroom (or wherever else you choose to get intimate)!

Chapter 7

Learning the Art of Oral Sex

Oral sex can be one of the most intimate and pleasurable experiences in the bedroom. It is an art form that requires skill, patience, and a willingness to explore new techniques and boundaries. If you want to drive your partner wild in bed, then learning the art of oral sex is key.

Different Types of Oral Sex

There are several different types of oral sex, including fellatio (oral sex on a man) and cunnilingus (oral sex on a woman). In addition, there are other variations that can be explored, such as rimming (oral stimulation of the anus) or tea bagging (placing testicles in the mouth).

How to Drive Him Wild in Bed

It's important to note that not everyone enjoys each type of oral sex, so communication with your partner is essential. Make sure to ask for their preferences and establish boundaries before engaging in any oral sex activities. Remember, you should never feel pressured to do something that you are not comfortable with.

Exploring Your and Your Partner's Boundaries

Before you can master the art of oral sex, you need to understand what works for you and your partner. Everyone is unique, so there is no one technique that will work for everyone. Take the time to explore each other's bodies and discover what feels good.

Start slowly and communicate often. Ask your partner what they like and don't like, and be open to feedback. Remember, this is a partnership, and both partners should be actively involved and engaged in the experience.

Tips for Mastering Different Techniques

Once you have established boundaries and taken the time to explore each other's bodies, you can start to experiment with different techniques.

Here are some tips for mastering different techniques:

Use your hands: Oral sex doesn't have to be limited to just your mouth. Try using your hands to stimulate your partner's erogenous zones while performing oral sex. Gently massage their body, kiss their neck, or fondle their genitals.

Pay attention to the clitoris: For women, the clitoris is the key to pleasure. It's important to understand that every woman is different and may enjoy different types of stimulation. Try different techniques such as gentle flicks or steady pressure to see what works best for your partner.

Don't forget about the balls: For men, the testicles are a highly sensitive area and can add another level of pleasure to oral sex. Be gentle and use only light pressure when stimulating this area.

Use your tongue creatively: Your tongue is one of the most versatile parts of your body and can be used in a variety of ways during oral sex. Try different techniques like lapping, swirling, flicking, or sucking to add variety and intensity.

Build up anticipation: Tease your partner by taking your time and building up anticipation. Kiss and stimulate other areas of their body before moving on to the genitals to increase the intensity of the experience.

Experiment with positions: Different oral sex positions can provide new sensations and make for a more pleasurable experience. You can try lying on your back with your head hanging off the edge of the bed, sitting on a chair or couch, or even standing up.

Communication is key: Always keep communication open throughout the entire experience. Check in with your partner regularly to gauge their level of enjoyment and adjust your techniques accordingly.

In conclusion, oral sex can be a highly pleasurable and intimate experience. The key to mastering this art is communication, exploration, and experimentation. Remember that every person is unique, so what works for one person may not work for another. Be open to feedback and willing to try new things.

Most importantly, always respect your partner's boundaries and stop immediately if either of you feel uncomfortable or unsafe. With patience, practice, and a little creativity, you can master the art of oral sex and create unforgettable erotic experiences that leave your partner begging for more.

How to Drive Him Wild in Bed

Chapter 8

Advanced Techniques for Driving Him Wild in Bed

Mastering Multiple Orgasms

Achieving multiple orgasms is a dream for many women, but did you know it's possible for men too? The key is to focus on the pleasure instead of the goal and embrace a mindset of exploration and experimentation. Start by exploring your own body and trying different techniques, such as edging or prostate stimulation. Then, involve your partner and communicate with them about what feels good during sex. By incorporating toys, role-playing or dirty talk, you can achieve multiple orgasms together and take your sexual connection to the next level.

How to Control Timing and Rhythm during Sex

Often times, timing and rhythm can make or break the experience in bed. One way to gain control over these factors is by practicing mindfulness and being fully present in the moment. Use your senses to guide you, focusing on your partner's body and the sensations you feel in your own. Experiment with different rhythms and tempos to find what works best for both of you. Also, don't forget to communicate with your partner and ask for feedback, as this will help you understand what they like and adjust your movements accordingly.

The Art of Teasing and Building Anticipation

Teasing and anticipation can be incredibly powerful tools for building arousal and intensifying pleasure. Start by setting the mood with candles, music, or a sexy outfit. Then, take your time with foreplay, exploring different erogenous zones and building anticipation before moving on to intercourse. Try using teasing techniques, such as tickling or nibbling, to heighten your partner's senses and get them worked up with desire. Another great way to build anticipation is through dirty talk. Whispering playful or seductive words and phrases into your partner's ear can be incredibly arousing and set the tone for a passionate encounter. But remember, building anticipation can be a delicate balance; you don't want to tease too much and leave your partner feeling unsatisfied, but you also don't want to give everything away too soon. The key is to pace yourself and follow your partner's lead.

Overall, mastering advanced techniques in the bedroom requires patience, practice, and a willingness to explore new sensations and experiences. By focusing on pleasure, communication, and building anticipation, you can take your sexual encounters to new heights of ecstasy and create unforgettable erotic experiences that leave both you and your partner begging for more.

Chapter 9

How to Create Unforgettable Erotic Experiences

Setting the Mood for a Passionate Night

One of the most important aspects of creating unforgettable erotic experiences is setting the right mood. This means creating an environment that is sensual and inviting, where both you and your partner feel comfortable and relaxed. Start by considering the details: lighting, music, scent, and temperature. Dim the lights or add candles, choose music that makes you feel confident and sexy, and use fragrance to create an ambiance. Consider also adding sensual fabrics, pillows, or bedding to your space for a luxurious touch. Taking the time to set the mood beforehand will help create an atmosphere that fosters intimacy and connection.

Creating a Sensual Environment in Your Bedroom

In addition to setting the mood, it's important to create a sensual environment in your bedroom to enhance the erotic experience. This can include incorporating items that stimulate the senses such as candles, incense, or aromatherapy. Consider investing in soft lighting fixtures such as dimmer switches or warm-colored bulbs. Add pillows and throws that emphasize the comfort and inviting nature of your bed. Finally, for an added touch, add some decorative elements that speak to your unique interests. Adding these personalized touches to your space can help create a sensory-rich environment that regulates anxiety and stress and promotes an extra layer of intimacy.

Dressing for Success

How you present yourself during sex plays a significant role in creating an unforgettable erotic experience. Generally, choosing attire that evokes your inner sexiness is essential for feeling confident and alluring. Consider selecting lingerie that accentuates the curve of your body and enhances your natural sex appeal.

Alternatively, opt for a silky or satin robe, sexy nightgown, or sleek bodycon dress to flatter your figure. Accessorize with statement jewelry or high heels to complete the look. Keep in mind, it's not just about how you look but also how you feel in your attire. Choose clothes that make you feel confident and empowered, as this energy will translate to the bedroom. Also, don't forget about your partner's preferences and consider wearing something that they find particularly alluring.

Ultimately, creating unforgettable erotic experiences is a mixture of setting the mood, creating a sensual environment, and dressing to impress. By incorporating these elements into your sexual routine, you can take your erotic encounters to the next level of pleasure and leave him begging for more.

Cheryl Bach

Chapter 10

How to Keep Him Begging for More

Communication is Key

To keep your lover begging for more, it's essential to maintain open communication about your sex life. This includes discussing your desires, likes, and dislikes, as well as any concerns or issues that arise. Take the time to understand your partner's needs and preferences, and communicate your own clearly and honestly. Additionally, make sure you express appreciation when something particularly pleasurable occurs. By keeping the lines of communication open, you can build a deeper level of trust and intimacy in your relationship, which will ultimately lead to greater pleasure.

Cheryl Bach

Fun and Interesting Sex Life

Routine sex can be exciting initially but soon becomes boring and monotonous. Keeping your sex life fun and interesting can help maintain the spark and keep your partner begging for more. Try experimenting with new positions, fantasies, or toys to add an exciting element to your routine. Additionally, consider planning surprises like role-playing or spontaneous encounters outside of the bedroom. By mixing things up and embracing new experiences, you can create a sexual relationship that remains fresh and exciting.

Incorporating New Techniques

Incorporating new techniques into your regular sex life can help keep things fresh and exciting. For instance, try practicing edging, where you bring yourself or your partner to the brink of orgasm and then stop. This can increase intensity and prolong pleasure in the long run. Another technique is Kama Sutra, which involves trying new positions that enhance pleasure. Tantra also involves incorporating mindfulness and meditation practices into your sexual routine. Experiment with different types of stimulation, such as erotic massage or using sex toys to explore new erogenous zones. By trying out new techniques and exploring different sensations, you can learn more about your body and your partner's, building a stronger connection and increasing pleasure.

Don't Be Afraid to Mix It Up

Sometimes the key to keeping your partner begging for more is to mix things up completely. Consider taking a romantic getaway to a new location, booking a hotel or spa stay, or creating a sensory deprivation situation for sex play. Try introducing an unexpected guest star in your routine, or setting up a game or challenge to add excitement and fun to your sexual encounters.

Cheryl Bach

In conclusion, to keep your partner begging for more, try adopting one or more of the above strategies to create a more intimate and varied sexual life. Remember that communication, fun, and experimentation are the keys to a healthy, fulfilling sexual relationship that leaves both you and your partner fully satisfied. Don't be afraid to mix things up, experiment with new techniques or toys, and keep things fun and lighthearted. The most important thing is to prioritize your partner's pleasure and show that you care for their sexual needs and desires. Keep an open mind, stay respectful, try something new each time, and enjoy all the unique and passionate erotic experiences that come your way. By following these tips, you'll become an expert at creating unforgettable erotic experiences that leave your partner begging for more. Good luck!

Chapter 11

Addressing Common Sexual Issues

Understanding and Overcoming Common Sexual Problems

Many couples experience common sexual issues such as performance anxiety, lack of desire, or erectile dysfunction. While it can be difficult to confront these issues, they are entirely normal and can affect people of all ages and genders. To overcome these problems, it is important to talk openly with your partner and find solutions that address your unique situation.

For performance anxiety, try practicing relaxation techniques such as deep breathing or meditation before sex. A positive mindset, realistic expectations, and focusing on the pleasure rather than the outcome may also help. For those experiencing a lack of desire, consider finding new ways to stimulate sexual curiosity, such as reading erotica together or exploring new fantasies. You might also prioritize self-care and reduce stress levels to help increase libido.

For those experiencing erectile dysfunction (ED), it is essential to understand that it can be caused by various factors, including physical or psychological issues. Consider seeking medical advice from a healthcare professional or a therapist who can help you address the underlying causes. There are also treatments available to help manage ED, such as medication or lifestyle changes. Remember, talking openly with your partner and seeking assistance when needed is key to overcoming common sexual problems.

Finding Help and Support for More Complex Sexual Issues

For more complex sexual issues, finding help and support can make all the difference. For instance, if you are experiencing intense sexual desires or urges that interfere with daily life, you might seek help from a licensed sex therapist or counselor who can help you develop coping strategies.

Additionally, some couples might struggle with differing levels of sexual desire or preferences. In this case, therapy or counseling can help couples communicate more effectively and address underlying resentment or lack of intimacy. It is important to remember that everyone has different sexual desires and needs, and there is no one-size-fits-all solution to these complex issues. However, finding qualified professionals who can help you work through these issues can be transformative and life-changing.

Another issue that may require professional help is if you or your partner have experienced sexual trauma or abuse. This can take a significant toll on mental health and physical wellbeing, and it is critical to seek therapy or counseling to overcome the trauma and find healing. In some cases, medication or psychiatry may also be recommended to address associated conditions like depression or anxiety.

Finally, it's important to remember that sexual preferences and gender are diverse and fluid, and may not fit neatly into societal norms or expectations. If you are struggling with gender identity or sexual orientation, reach out to community groups or LGBTQ+ resources for support and acceptance. Finding a supportive community and seeking therapy or counseling from experienced professionals can help you navigate the challenges that come with coming out or exploring your sexual identity.

Overall, addressing sexual issues requires a combination of openness with your partner, seeking help from professionals when needed, and being patient and compassionate with yourself. Remember that everyone experiences sexual problems at some point in their lives, and overcoming them is a normal part of any healthy sexual relationship. With the right mindset and support, you can work through these challenges and create a fulfilling and passionate sex life that satisfies both you and your partner.

Cheryl Bach

Chapter 12

Conclusion

Recap of the Key Points Covered in the Book

Throughout this book, we have covered a comprehensive guide to driving him wild in bed, mastering the art of passionate pleasure, and creating unforgettable erotic experiences that leave him begging for more. We've explored the importance of communication, experimentation, variety, and mutual satisfaction in achieving a fulfilling sexual relationship.

Here's a quick recap of some of the key points we've covered:

- Focus on communication and active listening to better understand your partner's desires and preferences

- Experiment with different techniques, positions, and environments to create exciting and unique experiences

- Prioritize mutual satisfaction by focusing on foreplay, practicing giving and receiving feedback, and being open to trying new things

- Explore your own desires and fantasies to bring more passion and excitement to your sexual encounters

- Push your boundaries and explore new areas of intimacy with your partner, always respecting each other's boundaries and comfort levels

- Keep things fun and lighthearted by maintaining a playful attitude and not taking yourselves too seriously

Remember that sex is not just a physical act, but a mental and emotional experience as well. Prioritize intimacy and emotional connection to make your sexual encounters more fulfilling.

Encouragement to Continue Exploring Sexual Pleasure with Your Partner

It's important to remember that sexual exploration and pleasure is a lifelong journey, and it's never too late to start experiencing new things with your partner. Whether you've been together for weeks, months, or years, there's always room for growth, experimentation, and increased satisfaction in your sexual relationship.

By prioritizing communication, mutual satisfaction, and open-mindedness, you can continue to explore new areas of intimacy and pleasure with your partner, deepening your emotional connection and creating unforgettable erotic experiences together. It's okay to take things slow and to start small, focusing on building trust and comfort with each other as you explore new territories of intimacy at a pace that feels right for both of you.

Cheryl Bach

So go ahead and experiment with different techniques, try new positions, explore your own desires and fantasies and communicate with your partner to uncover his as well. Create an environment of trust and openness, be willing to take risks and embrace what you both love to do together.

Remember that sexual pleasure is a journey – not a destination. So keep exploring, stay open to new experiences, and most importantly, have fun with it! With the right mindset and techniques, you can create a sex life that's fulfilling, adventurous, and beyond anything you've ever imagined. Good luck and enjoy your exploration together!